# This journal belongs to

_____

_____

_____

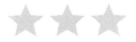

# The 5 rules to create positive affirmations

- Always start with "I" or "My"

- Always use the present tense: say "I am" or "I feel" but not "I will" or "I should"

- Never use negations: say "I always succeed" and not "I never fail"

- Be precise and concise: don't say "I'm grateful" but "I'm grateful for having two awesome children"

- Always include a feeling

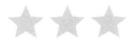

# 10 examples of positive affirmations

- My life is a joy filled with love, fun and friendship
- I'm a do-er : I take action and get things accomplished
- I finish every thing I start
- I'm responsible for everything happening in my life
- The universe provides for my every want and need
- I believe in my skills and abilities
- My body is a temple. I will keep my temple clean
- I make positive healthy choices
- I search for the good that comes even in bad situations
- I am so grateful for my life

# Date    M T W T F S S

## One goal for today

_____

_____

## Today's positive affirmation

_____

_____

_____

_____

## My thoughts for today

_____

_____

_____

_____

_____

## My mood today

★ ★ ★ ★ ★ ★ ★ ★ ★ ★

# Did I stay sober today?

## YES          NO

# Was today's goal accomplished?

## YES          NO

# What I am grateful for today

_____

_____

_____

# What I am proud of today

_____

_____

_____

# My plans for tomorrow

_____

_____

# Date  M T W T F S S

## One goal for today

## Today's positive affirmation

## My thoughts for today

## My mood today

# Did I stay sober today?

### YES          NO

# Was today's goal accomplished?

### YES          NO

# What I am grateful for today

_____

_____

_____

# What I am proud of today

_____

_____

_____

# My plans for tomorrow

_____

_____

_____

# Date        M T W T F S S

## One goal for today

_____

_____

## Today's positive affirmation

_____

_____

_____

## My thoughts for today

_____

_____

_____

_____

_____

## My mood today

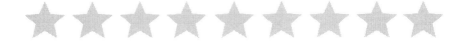

# Did I stay sober today?

## YES     NO

# Was today's goal accomplished?

## YES     NO

# What I am grateful for today

_____

_____

_____

# What I am proud of today

_____

_____

_____

# My plans for tomorrow

_____

_____

_____

# Date          M T W T F S S

## One goal for today

_____

## Today's positive affirmation

_____

_____

## My thoughts for today

_____

_____

_____

## My mood today

★ ★ ★ ★ ★ ★ ★ ★ ★ ★

# Did I stay sober today?

## YES    NO

# Was today's goal accomplished?

## YES    NO

# What I am grateful for today

_____

_____

_____

# What I am proud of today

_____

_____

_____

# My plans for tomorrow

_____

_____

_____

# Date     M T W T F S S

## One goal for today

---

## Today's positive affirmation

---

---

---

## My thoughts for today

---

---

---

---

## My mood today

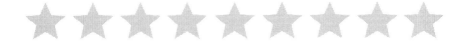

# Did I stay sober today?

YES          NO

# Was today's goal accomplished?

YES          NO

# What I am grateful for today

_____

_____

_____

# What I am proud of today

_____

_____

_____

# My plans for tomorrow

_____

_____

_____

# Date     M T W T F S S

## One goal for today

## Today's positive affirmation

## My thoughts for today

## My mood today

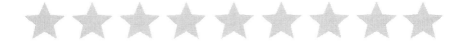

# Did I stay sober today?

### YES    NO

# Was today's goal accomplished?

### YES    NO

# What I am grateful for today

_____

_____

_____

# What I am proud of today

_____

_____

_____

# My plans for tomorrow

_____

_____

_____

# Date        M T W T F S S

## One goal for today

## Today's positive affirmation

## My thoughts for today

## My mood today

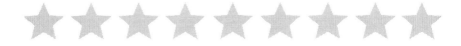

# Did I stay sober today?

YES      NO

# Was today's goal accomplished?

YES      NO

# What I am grateful for today

_____

_____

_____

# What I am proud of today

_____

_____

_____

# My plans for tomorrow

_____

_____

_____

# Date        M T W T F S S

## One goal for today

_____

_____

## Today's positive affirmation

_____

_____

_____

## My thoughts for today

_____

_____

_____

_____

## My mood today

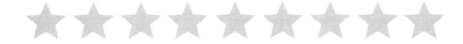

# Did I stay sober today?

## YES     NO

# Was today's goal accomplished?

## YES     NO

# What I am grateful for today

_____

_____

_____

# What I am proud of today

_____

_____

_____

# My plans for tomorrow

_____

_____

# Date      M T W T F S S

## One goal for today

_____

_____

## Today's positive affirmation

_____

_____

_____

## My thoughts for today

_____

_____

_____

_____

## My mood today

⭐ ⭐ ⭐ ⭐ ⭐ ⭐ ⭐ ⭐ ⭐ ⭐

# Did I stay sober today?

YES     NO

# Was today's goal accomplished?

YES     NO

# What I am grateful for today

_____

_____

_____

# What I am proud of today

_____

_____

_____

# My plans for tomorrow

_____

_____

_____

# Date M T W T F S S

## One goal for today

---

---

## Today's positive affirmation

---

---

---

---

## My thoughts for today

---

---

---

---

---

## My mood today

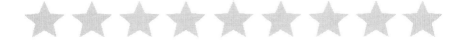

# Did I stay sober today?

## YES      NO

# Was today's goal accomplished?

## YES      NO

# What I am grateful for today

_____

_____

_____

# What I am proud of today

_____

_____

_____

# My plans for tomorrow

_____

_____

# Date    M T W T F S S

## One goal for today

## Today's positive affirmation

## My thoughts for today

## My mood today

★ ★ ★ ★ ★ ★ ★ ★ ★ ★

# Did I stay sober today?

YES       NO

# Was today's goal accomplished?

YES       NO

# What I am grateful for today

_____

_____

_____

# What I am proud of today

_____

_____

_____

# My plans for tomorrow

_____

_____

_____

# Date      M T W T F S S

## One goal for today

_____

## Today's positive affirmation

_____

_____

## My thoughts for today

_____

_____

_____

## My mood today

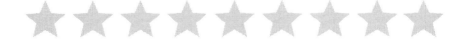

# Did I stay sober today?

### YES     NO

# Was today's goal accomplished?

### YES     NO

# What I am grateful for today

_____

_____

_____

# What I am proud of today

_____

_____

_____

# My plans for tomorrow

_____

_____

_____

# Date    M T W T F S S

## One goal for today

_____

_____

## Today's positive affirmation

_____

_____

_____

## My thoughts for today

_____

_____

_____

_____

## My mood today

★ ★ ★ ★ ★ ★ ★ ★ ★ ★

# Did I stay sober today?

### YES      NO

# Was today's goal accomplished?

### YES      NO

# What I am grateful for today

_____

_____

_____

# What I am proud of today

_____

_____

_____

# My plans for tomorrow

_____

_____

_____

# Date     M T W T F S S

## One goal for today

_____

_____

## Today's positive affirmation

_____

_____

_____

## My thoughts for today

_____

_____

_____

_____

## My mood today

★ ★ ★ ★ ★ ★ ★ ★ ★ ★

# Did I stay sober today?

## YES      NO

# Was today's goal accomplished?

## YES      NO

# What I am grateful for today

_____

_____

_____

# What I am proud of today

_____

_____

_____

# My plans for tomorrow

_____

_____

_____

# Date     M T W T F S S

## One goal for today

## Today's positive affirmation

## My thoughts for today

## My mood today

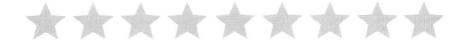

# Did I stay sober today?

## YES        NO

# Was today's goal accomplished?

## YES        NO

# What I am grateful for today

_____

_____

_____

# What I am proud of today

_____

_____

_____

# My plans for tomorrow

_____

_____

_____

# Date          M T W T F S S

## One goal for today

_____

_____

## Today's positive affirmation

_____

_____

_____

## My thoughts for today

_____

_____

_____

_____

## My mood today

★ ★ ★ ★ ★ ★ ★ ★ ★ ★

# Did I stay sober today?

YES     NO

# Was today's goal accomplished?

YES     NO

# What I am grateful for today

_____

_____

_____

# What I am proud of today

_____

_____

_____

# My plans for tomorrow

_____

_____

_____

# Date    M T W T F S S

## One goal for today

---

## Today's positive affirmation

---

---

## My thoughts for today

---

---

---

## My mood today

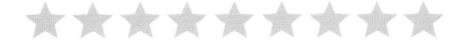

# Did I stay sober today?

## YES     NO

# Was today's goal accomplished?

## YES     NO

# What I am grateful for today

_____

_____

_____

# What I am proud of today

_____

_____

_____

# My plans for tomorrow

_____

_____

# Date      M T W T F S S

## One goal for today

## Today's positive affirmation

## My thoughts for today

## My mood today

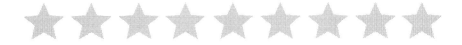

# Did I stay sober today?

## YES    NO

# Was today's goal accomplished?

## YES    NO

# What I am grateful for today

_____

_____

_____

# What I am proud of today

_____

_____

_____

# My plans for tomorrow

_____

_____

_____

# Date　　MTWTFSS

## One goal for today

_____

_____

## Today's positive affirmation

_____

_____

_____

## My thoughts for today

_____

_____

_____

_____

## My mood today

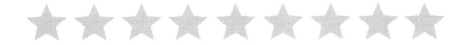

# Did I stay sober today?

## YES     NO

# Was today's goal accomplished?

## YES     NO

# What I am grateful for today

_____

_____

_____

# What I am proud of today

_____

_____

_____

# My plans for tomorrow

_____

_____

_____

# Date     M T W T F S S

## One goal for today

## Today's positive affirmation

## My thoughts for today

## My mood today

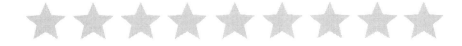

# Did I stay sober today?

## YES     NO

# Was today's goal accomplished?

## YES     NO

# What I am grateful for today

_____

_____

_____

_____

# What I am proud of today

_____

_____

_____

# My plans for tomorrow

_____

_____

_____

# Date　　　M T W T F S S

## One goal for today

## Today's positive affirmation

## My thoughts for today

## My mood today

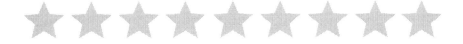

# Did I stay sober today?

YES     NO

# Was today's goal accomplished?

YES     NO

# What I am grateful for today

_____

_____

_____

# What I am proud of today

_____

_____

_____

# My plans for tomorrow

_____

_____

_____

# Date     M T W T F S S

## One goal for today

---

---

## Today's positive affirmation

---

---

---

---

## My thoughts for today

---

---

---

---

## My mood today

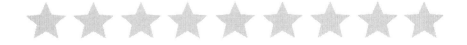

# Did I stay sober today?

## YES      NO

# Was today's goal accomplished?

## YES      NO

# What I am grateful for today

_____

_____

_____

# What I am proud of today

_____

_____

_____

# My plans for tomorrow

_____

_____

_____

# Date     M T W T F S S

## One goal for today

_____

_____

## Today's positive affirmation

_____

_____

_____

## My thoughts for today

_____

_____

_____

_____

## My mood today

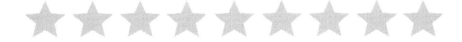

# Did I stay sober today?

YES     NO

# Was today's goal accomplished?

YES     NO

# What I am grateful for today

_____

_____

_____

# What I am proud of today

_____

_____

_____

# My plans for tomorrow

_____

_____

_____

# Date    M T W T F S S

## One goal for today

## Today's positive affirmation

## My thoughts for today

## My mood today

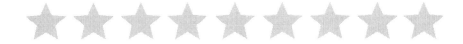

# Did I stay sober today?

## YES     NO

# Was today's goal accomplished?

## YES     NO

# What I am grateful for today

_____

_____

_____

# What I am proud of today

_____

_____

_____

# My plans for tomorrow

_____

_____

_____

# Date　　　M T W T F S S

## One goal for today

## Today's positive affirmation

## My thoughts for today

## My mood today

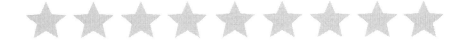

# Did I stay sober today?

### YES     NO

# Was today's goal accomplished?

### YES     NO

# What I am grateful for today

_____

_____

_____

# What I am proud of today

_____

_____

_____

# My plans for tomorrow

_____

_____

_____

# Date          M T W T F S S

## One goal for today

## Today's positive affirmation

## My thoughts for today

## My mood today

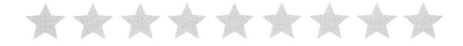

# Did I stay sober today?

## YES        NO

# Was today's goal accomplished?

## YES        NO

# What I am grateful for today

_____

_____

_____

_____

# What I am proud of today

_____

_____

_____

# My plans for tomorrow

_____

_____

_____

# Date     M T W T F S S

## One goal for today

_____

_____

## Today's positive affirmation

_____

_____

_____

## My thoughts for today

_____

_____

_____

_____

## My mood today

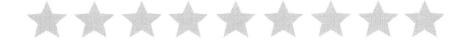

# Did I stay sober today?

## YES    NO

# Was today's goal accomplished?

## YES    NO

# What I am grateful for today

_____

_____

_____

# What I am proud of today

_____

_____

_____

# My plans for tomorrow

_____

_____

_____

# Date     M T W T F S S

## One goal for today

## Today's positive affirmation

## My thoughts for today

## My mood today

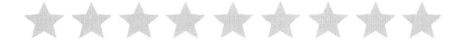

# Did I stay sober today?

### YES      NO

# Was today's goal accomplished?

### YES      NO

# What I am grateful for today

_____

_____

_____

# What I am proud of today

_____

_____

_____

# My plans for tomorrow

_____

_____

_____

# Date   M T W T F S S

## One goal for today

## Today's positive affirmation

## My thoughts for today

## My mood today

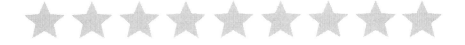

# Did I stay sober today?

## YES     NO

# Was today's goal accomplished?

## YES     NO

# What I am grateful for today

_____

_____

_____

_____

# What I am proud of today

_____

_____

_____

# My plans for tomorrow

_____

_____

_____

# Date  M T W T F S S

## One goal for today

_____

_____

## Today's positive affirmation

_____

_____

_____

## My thoughts for today

_____

_____

_____

_____

## My mood today

★ ★ ★ ★ ★ ★ ★ ★ ★ ★

# Did I stay sober today?

YES      NO

# Was today's goal accomplished?

YES      NO

# What I am grateful for today

_____

_____

_____

# What I am proud of today

_____

_____

_____

# My plans for tomorrow

_____

_____

_____

# Date      M T W T F S S

## One goal for today

## Today's positive affirmation

## My thoughts for today

## My mood today

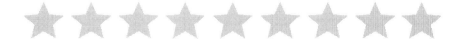

# Did I stay sober today?

YES          NO

# Was today's goal accomplished?

YES          NO

# What I am grateful for today

_____

_____

_____

# What I am proud of today

_____

_____

_____

# My plans for tomorrow

_____

_____

_____

# Date     M T W T F S S

## One goal for today

_____

## Today's positive affirmation

_____

_____

_____

## My thoughts for today

_____

_____

_____

_____

## My mood today

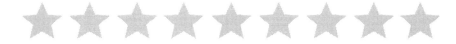

# Did I stay sober today?

## YES        NO

# Was today's goal accomplished?

## YES        NO

# What I am grateful for today

_____

_____

_____

# What I am proud of today

_____

_____

_____

# My plans for tomorrow

_____

_____

_____

# Date     M T W T F S S

## One goal for today

_____

## Today's positive affirmation

_____

_____

## My thoughts for today

_____

_____

_____

## My mood today

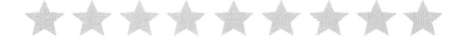

# Did I stay sober today?

YES      NO

# Was today's goal accomplished?

YES      NO

# What I am grateful for today

_____

_____

_____

# What I am proud of today

_____

_____

_____

# My plans for tomorrow

_____

_____

_____

# Date    M T W T F S S

## One goal for today

## Today's positive affirmation

## My thoughts for today

## My mood today

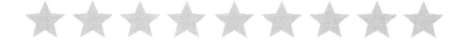

# Did I stay sober today?

YES     NO

# Was today's goal accomplished?

YES     NO

# What I am grateful for today

_____

_____

_____

_____

# What I am proud of today

_____

_____

_____

# My plans for tomorrow

_____

_____

_____

# Date     M T W T F S S

## One goal for today

---

---

## Today's positive affirmation

---

---

---

## My thoughts for today

---

---

---

---

## My mood today

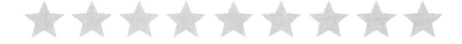

# Did I stay sober today?

YES      NO

# Was today's goal accomplished?

YES      NO

# What I am grateful for today

_____

_____

_____

# What I am proud of today

_____

_____

_____

# My plans for tomorrow

_____

_____

_____

# Date     M T W T F S S

## One goal for today

## Today's positive affirmation

## My thoughts for today

## My mood today

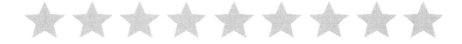

# Did I stay sober today?

YES      NO

# Was today's goal accomplished?

YES      NO

# What I am grateful for today

_____

_____

_____

# What I am proud of today

_____

_____

_____

# My plans for tomorrow

_____

_____

_____

# Date     M T W T F S S

## One goal for today

---

## Today's positive affirmation

---

## My thoughts for today

---

## My mood today

★ ★ ★ ★ ★ ★ ★ ★ ★ ★

# Did I stay sober today?

YES     NO

# Was today's goal accomplished?

YES     NO

# What I am grateful for today

_____

_____

_____

# What I am proud of today

_____

_____

_____

# My plans for tomorrow

_____

_____

_____

# Date    M T W T F S S

## One goal for today

_____

_____

## Today's positive affirmation

_____

_____

_____

## My thoughts for today

_____

_____

_____

_____

_____

## My mood today

★ ★ ★ ★ ★ ★ ★ ★ ★ ★

# Did I stay sober today?

YES        NO

# Was today's goal accomplished?

YES        NO

# What I am grateful for today

_____

_____

_____

_____

# What I am proud of today

_____

_____

_____

# My plans for tomorrow

_____

_____

_____

# Date      M T W T F S S

## One goal for today

## Today's positive affirmation

## My thoughts for today

## My mood today

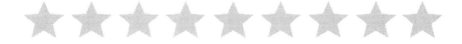

# Did I stay sober today?

YES     NO

# Was today's goal accomplished?

YES     NO

# What I am grateful for today

_____

_____

_____

# What I am proud of today

_____

_____

_____

# My plans for tomorrow

_____

_____

_____

# Date        M T W T F S S

## One goal for today

_____

## Today's positive affirmation

_____

_____

## My thoughts for today

_____

_____

_____

## My mood today

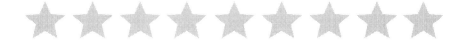

# Did I stay sober today?

YES     NO

# Was today's goal accomplished?

YES     NO

# What I am grateful for today

_____

_____

_____

# What I am proud of today

_____

_____

_____

# My plans for tomorrow

_____

_____

_____

# Date        M T W T F S S

## One goal for today

_____

## Today's positive affirmation

_____

_____

_____

## My thoughts for today

_____

_____

_____

_____

## My mood today

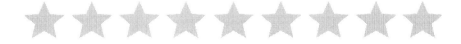

Did I stay sober today?

YES       NO

Was today's goal accomplished?

YES       NO

What I am grateful for today

_____

_____

_____

What I am proud of today

_____

_____

_____

My plans for tomorrow

_____

_____

_____

# Date       M T W T F S S

## One goal for today

## Today's positive affirmation

## My thoughts for today

## My mood today

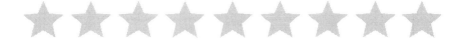

# Did I stay sober today?

## YES   NO

# Was today's goal accomplished?

## YES   NO

# What I am grateful for today

_____

_____

_____

# What I am proud of today

_____

_____

_____

# My plans for tomorrow

_____

_____

_____

# Date     M T W T F S S

## One goal for today

_____

_____

## Today's positive affirmation

_____

_____

_____

## My thoughts for today

_____

_____

_____

_____

## My mood today

★ ★ ★ ★ ★ ★ ★ ★ ★ ★

# Did I stay sober today?

YES      NO

# Was today's goal accomplished?

YES      NO

# What I am grateful for today

_____

_____

_____

# What I am proud of today

_____

_____

_____

# My plans for tomorrow

_____

_____

_____

# Date  M T W T F S S

## One goal for today

_____

## Today's positive affirmation

_____

_____

## My thoughts for today

_____

_____

_____

## My mood today

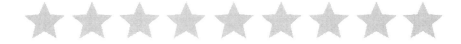

# Did I stay sober today?

## YES      NO

# Was today's goal accomplished?

## YES      NO

# What I am grateful for today

_____

_____

_____

# What I am proud of today

_____

_____

_____

# My plans for tomorrow

_____

_____

_____

# Date       M T W T F S S

## One goal for today

_____

_____

## Today's positive affirmation

_____

_____

_____

## My thoughts for today

_____

_____

_____

_____

_____

## My mood today

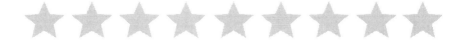

# Did I stay sober today?

YES     NO

# Was today's goal accomplished?

YES     NO

# What I am grateful for today

_____

_____

_____

# What I am proud of today

_____

_____

_____

# My plans for tomorrow

_____

_____

_____

# Date     M T W T F S S

## One goal for today

_____

## Today's positive affirmation

_____

_____

## My thoughts for today

_____

_____

_____

_____

## My mood today

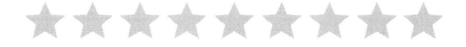

# Did I stay sober today?

YES     NO

# Was today's goal accomplished?

YES     NO

# What I am grateful for today

_____

_____

_____

# What I am proud of today

_____

_____

_____

# My plans for tomorrow

_____

_____

_____

# Date          M T W T F S S

## One goal for today

_____

_____

## Today's positive affirmation

_____

_____

_____

## My thoughts for today

_____

_____

_____

_____

## My mood today

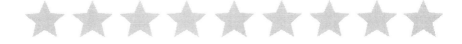

# Did I stay sober today?

YES     NO

# Was today's goal accomplished?

YES     NO

# What I am grateful for today

_____

_____

_____

# What I am proud of today

_____

_____

_____

# My plans for tomorrow

_____

_____

_____

# Date     M T W T F S S

## One goal for today

_____

_____

## Today's positive affirmation

_____

_____

_____

## My thoughts for today

_____

_____

_____

_____

## My mood today

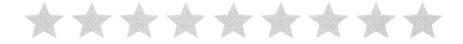

# Did I stay sober today?

## YES     NO

# Was today's goal accomplished?

## YES     NO

# What I am grateful for today

_____

_____

_____

_____

# What I am proud of today

_____

_____

_____

# My plans for tomorrow

_____

_____

_____

# Date  M T W T F S S

## One goal for today

_____

## Today's positive affirmation

_____

_____

_____

## My thoughts for today

_____

_____

_____

_____

## My mood today

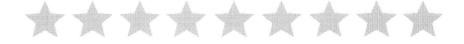

# Did I stay sober today?

## YES    NO

# Was today's goal accomplished?

## YES    NO

# What I am grateful for today

_____

_____

_____

_____

# What I am proud of today

_____

_____

_____

# My plans for tomorrow

_____

_____

_____

# Date     M T W T F S S

## One goal for today

## Today's positive affirmation

## My thoughts for today

## My mood today

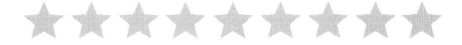

# Did I stay sober today?

YES     NO

## Was today's goal accomplished?

YES     NO

## What I am grateful for today

_____

_____

_____

## What I am proud of today

_____

_____

_____

## My plans for tomorrow

_____

_____

# Date     M T W T F S S

## One goal for today

_____

_____

## Today's positive affirmation

_____

_____

_____

## My thoughts for today

_____

_____

_____

_____

## My mood today

★ ★ ★ ★ ★ ★ ★ ★ ★ ★

# Did I stay sober today?

YES     NO

# Was today's goal accomplished?

YES     NO

# What I am grateful for today

_____

_____

_____

# What I am proud of today

_____

_____

_____

# My plans for tomorrow

_____

_____

_____

# Date          M T W T F S S

## One goal for today

_____

## Today's positive affirmation

_____

_____

_____

## My thoughts for today

_____

_____

_____

_____

## My mood today

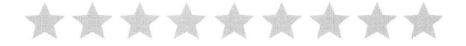

# Did I stay sober today?

YES     NO

# Was today's goal accomplished?

YES     NO

# What I am grateful for today

_____

_____

_____

# What I am proud of today

_____

_____

_____

# My plans for tomorrow

_____

_____

_____

# Date  M T W T F S S

## One goal for today

## Today's positive affirmation

## My thoughts for today

## My mood today

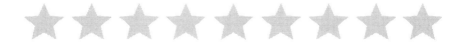

# Did I stay sober today?

## YES    NO

# Was today's goal accomplished?

## YES    NO

# What I am grateful for today

_____

_____

_____

_____

# What I am proud of today

_____

_____

_____

# My plans for tomorrow

_____

_____

_____

# Date     M T W T F S S

## One goal for today

_____

_____

## Today's positive affirmation

_____

_____

_____

_____

## My thoughts for today

_____

_____

_____

_____

_____

## My mood today

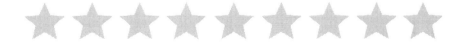

# Did I stay sober today?

### YES     NO

# Was today's goal accomplished?

### YES     NO

# What I am grateful for today

_____

_____

_____

_____

# What I am proud of today

_____

_____

_____

# My plans for tomorrow

_____

_____

_____

# Date       M T W T F S S

## One goal for today

_____

_____

## Today's positive affirmation

_____

_____

_____

_____

## My thoughts for today

_____

_____

_____

_____

## My mood today

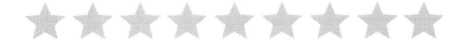

# Did I stay sober today?

### YES    NO

# Was today's goal accomplished?

### YES    NO

# What I am grateful for today

_____

_____

_____

# What I am proud of today

_____

_____

_____

# My plans for tomorrow

_____

_____

# Date    M T W T F S S

## One goal for today

---

## Today's positive affirmation

---

---

---

## My thoughts for today

---

---

---

---

## My mood today

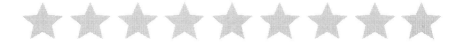

# Did I stay sober today?

YES          NO

# Was today's goal accomplished?

YES          NO

# What I am grateful for today

_____

_____

_____

# What I am proud of today

_____

_____

_____

# My plans for tomorrow

_____

_____

_____

# Date     M T W T F S S

## One goal for today

---

## Today's positive affirmation

---

## My thoughts for today

---

## My mood today

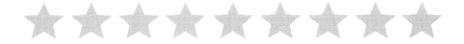

# Did I stay sober today?

### YES          NO

# Was today's goal accomplished?

### YES          NO

# What I am grateful for today

_____

_____

_____

# What I am proud of today

_____

_____

# My plans for tomorrow

_____

_____

# Date     M T W T F S S

## One goal for today

## Today's positive affirmation

## My thoughts for today

## My mood today

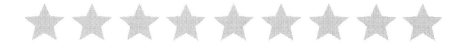

# Did I stay sober today?

YES        NO

# Was today's goal accomplished?

YES        NO

# What I am grateful for today

_____

_____

_____

# What I am proud of today

_____

_____

_____

# My plans for tomorrow

_____

_____

# Date          M T W T F S S

## One goal for today

## Today's positive affirmation

## My thoughts for today

## My mood today

# Did I stay sober today?

## YES        NO

# Was today's goal accomplished?

## YES        NO

# What I am grateful for today

_____

_____

_____

# What I am proud of today

_____

_____

_____

# My plans for tomorrow

_____

_____

_____

# Date          M T W T F S S

## One goal for today

_____

_____

## Today's positive affirmation

_____

_____

_____

## My thoughts for today

_____

_____

_____

_____

_____

## My mood today

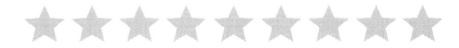

# Did I stay sober today?

## YES    NO

# Was today's goal accomplished?

## YES    NO

# What I am grateful for today

_____

_____

_____

# What I am proud of today

_____

_____

_____

# My plans for tomorrow

_____

_____

26239261R00073

Printed in Great Britain
by Amazon